The Logic of Healing:
Understanding the Choices, Timing, and Stories Behind Your Treatment

By Dr. SALEEM AKRAM (Pharmacist Pharm D)

Disclaimer:

This book is intended for educational and informational purposes only. It is not a substitute for professional medical advice, diagnosis, or treatment. Readers should not use the information in this book to make medical decisions without consulting a qualified healthcare professional.

The author makes no representations or warranties regarding the accuracy or completeness of the information provided and assumes no liability for its use.

The stories and case examples presented in this book are fictional. Any resemblance to actual persons, living or dead, or to real events is coincidental and used solely for illustrative and educational purposes.

Dedication

This book is dedicated to my mentors the teachers who shaped my understanding of science, the guides who taught me how to think with care, and the voices who reminded me that knowledge carries responsibility.

Your patience, rigor, and belief in thoughtful communication shaped not only my training, but my approach to healthcare itself. Every chapter in this book carries the influence of what you taught me: that medicine is not only about knowing more, but about explaining better.

Table of Contents

PREFACE

This book began with a simple and persistent observation: most people want to follow their doctor's instructions, yet many struggle to understand the reasoning behind them.

Across clinics, pharmacies, and everyday conversations, I encountered the same quiet pattern. Patients were doing their best to follow treatment plans. Clinicians were doing their best to provide care. And still, a gap remained between what was prescribed and what was practiced. Not because of negligence or defiance, but because understanding often stopped at the surface.

My training as a pharmacist taught me how medicines work, how the body responds to illness, and how treatment plans are constructed. But my work beyond the clinic in writing, editing, and publishing taught me something equally important: information alone does not create understanding. Knowledge becomes meaningful only when it is communicated clearly, patiently, and in a way that respects how people actually live.

Too often, medical instructions are delivered without the story behind them. Patients are told what to do, but not why it matters. When the reasoning remains hidden, instructions can feel rigid, optional, or disconnected from real life. In that space, uncertainty grows and with it, hesitation, adjustment, or abandonment of treatment plans.

This book is not a medical manual, and it is not a guide to self-treatment. It does not tell readers what decisions to make. Instead, it explores how medical decisions are made in the first place. It explains how clinicians think, why details matter, and how small choices can influence outcomes in ways that are not always obvious.

Every chapter is written with a single intention: to replace confusion with clarity, and to replace silent doubt with understanding. The stories in this book are fictional, but they are shaped by real experiences familiar to anyone who has navigated illness, uncertainty, or the complexity of healthcare.

If this book helps even one reader feel more informed, more confident, or more engaged in their care, it has served its purpose. And if it encourages more open conversations between patients and healthcare professionals, then it has done something even more important.

A Note to the Reader

How to Read This Book

This book is not meant to be read as a set of instructions, nor as a substitute for medical advice. It does not tell you what decisions to make about your health. Instead, it explains how medical decisions are made, and why the instructions that follow them are often misunderstood.

You may choose to read this book straight through, and it will reward that approach. The chapters build logically, moving from the foundations of clinical reasoning to the points where understanding most commonly breaks down. Taken together, they form a coherent picture of how treatment plans are designed and how they interact with real lives.

You may also find yourself returning to specific sections as questions arise. The chapters in Part II, which explore common misinterpretations, are written to stand on their own. They reflect moments many patients recognize times when improvement feels like permission to stop, discomfort feels like failure, or caution feels like safety. If a particular belief resonates with your experience, you can begin there.

Throughout the book, you will encounter fictional cases. These stories are not meant to represent extreme situations or unusual patients. They are intentionally ordinary. Their purpose is not to dramatize illness, but to show how reasonable people think through uncertainty when context is incomplete. If you recognize yourself in these stories, that recognition is the point.

This book assumes good faith on all sides. Patients are not portrayed as careless, and clinicians are not portrayed as infallible. Healthcare works best when both perspectives are understood and respected. The aim here is not compliance, but clarity; not authority, but alignment.

If you are a patient, this book is meant to help you interpret medical guidance more confidently and communicate more effectively with those who care for you. If you are a clinician, it may offer language and perspective for conversations you already know are difficult to compress into short visits. If you are a caregiver or family member, it may help you understand the reasoning behind plans that can otherwise feel opaque.

You do not need to agree with every decision described here. You do not need to follow every example. What matters is understanding the framework behind them. When that framework is clear, questions become more precise, conversations more productive, and decisions more deliberate.

This book is not about certainty. Medicine rarely offers that. It is about reasoning, partnership, and the shared responsibility of understanding. Read it at your own pace, return to it when needed, and use it as a lens not a rulebook.

Introduction: The Gap Between Prescription and Practice

Most people recognize the moment. You leave a doctor's office with clear instructions in hand, yet a quiet hesitation follows you out the door. The prescription makes sense in theory, but life is busy. Symptoms fluctuate. And somewhere between intention and routine, the question arises: Do I really need to follow this exactly as written?

That hesitation is rarely spoken aloud, yet it is nearly universal. It appears in kitchens where pills are placed beside breakfast and forgotten by lunchtime. In bedrooms where alarms are set with good intentions and silenced without thought. In workplaces where schedules collide with routines. This is where treatment plans succeed or falter not because people do not care, but because the reasoning behind those plans is often invisible.

Medical care does not end at the clinic door. It continues in everyday life, where decisions are shaped by habits, emotions, and practical constraints. When patients do not understand why instructions are designed a certain way, it becomes easier to modify them skip a dose, change the timing, stop early without realizing the consequences.

Doctors and pharmacists spend years learning how illnesses behave and how treatments interact with the body. Patients, meanwhile, are asked to trust instructions that can feel overly precise or unnecessarily strict. When the logic behind those instructions is unclear, uncertainty fills the gap. And uncertainty quietly influences choices.

Understanding medical reasoning does not require a medical degree. It requires curiosity and context. Behind every prescription is a series of decisions shaped by biology, risk, and experience. When a doctor recommends a specific medication, dose, or schedule, there is a reason often rooted in how the body works and how small details affect outcomes.

This book brings those reasons into view.

It does not offer shortcuts or alternatives. It does not replace professional advice. Instead, it explains the principles that guide medical decisions, the trade-offs clinicians weigh, and the logic behind the instructions patients receive. By understanding these foundations, patients can approach their treatment plans with greater clarity and confidence.

The chapters that follow explore how prescribing decisions are made, why dosing and timing matter, how adherence affects outcomes, and how human psychology shapes health behavior. Through realistic, fictional stories, we will examine how misunderstandings arise and how clarity restores balance.

At its core, this book is about partnership. Medical care is not a one-sided exchange of instructions. It is a shared effort between those who understand the science and those who live with its application. When both sides understand each other more fully, treatment becomes less about rules and more about collaboration.

Understanding closes the gap between prescription and practice. And understanding is where healing begins.

PART I Foundations of Medical Reasoning

Most interactions with healthcare begin at the surface. A symptom is described, a diagnosis considered, a prescription written, instructions given. From the patient's perspective, this sequence can feel linear and transactional an exchange of information followed by a set of expectations. What often remains unseen is the depth of reasoning beneath those expectations.

Medical decisions are rarely simple, even when they appear so. Behind every prescription lies a network of considerations: how the body functions, how illness behaves over time, how treatments interact with existing conditions, and how real lives complicate ideal plans. These considerations are not always articulated, not because they are unimportant, but because they are assumed to be understood or too complex to explain in limited time.

This assumption creates a gap.

Patients are asked to carry out instructions shaped by logic they have not been invited into. Clinicians, trained to think in probabilities, systems, and timelines, often underestimate how unfamiliar this reasoning can feel outside the clinical context. The result is not mistrust, but misalignment between what is intended and what is understood.

This first section makes that hidden reasoning visible.

The chapters that follow explore how clinicians think before a treatment plan ever reaches the patient. They examine why dosing is precise, why timing matters, why consistency is emphasized, and why deviation however reasonable it may seem can alter outcomes. They also consider the psychological realities that influence how instructions are received, interpreted, and acted upon.

This is not a guide to self-treatment, nor a manual for medical decision-making. It is an invitation into the logic that underpins care. By understanding how and why decisions are made, patients are better equipped to engage with them not as passive recipients, but as informed participants.

The goal of this section is not agreement, but context. When people understand the framework behind medical guidance, questions become more precise, conversations more productive, and decisions more deliberate. Understanding does not eliminate uncertainty, but it reduces confusion. It transforms instructions from rigid rules into reasoned recommendations.

Before examining where misunderstanding arises, it is necessary to understand what is being misunderstood. This section lays that groundwork. It explains the architecture of medical reasoning not in technical terms, but in human ones.

What follows is the logic of care as it is practiced, not as it is often perceived.

Chapter 1: What Doctors Really Consider Before Prescribing

On a rainy Tuesday afternoon, Farid sat across from his doctor, describing a dull ache that had settled into his lower back weeks earlier. He expected a brief exchange and a straightforward solution perhaps a strong pain reliever or a muscle relaxant. Instead, the appointment unfolded differently. The doctor asked about the pain's duration, what made it better or worse, Farid's sleep patterns, his daily routine, and the medications he took regularly. Then came questions that seemed even less connected: kidney health, previous injuries, work stress, and how often he exercised.

Farid answered patiently, though with growing confusion. To him, the problem felt simple. His back hurt. Why did solving it require so many questions?

What Farid could not see was the quiet process taking shape beneath the surface. As he spoke, the doctor was not searching for a single diagnosis or a quick fix. She was building a mental framework an internal map shaped by medical knowledge, clinical experience, and an understanding of how different factors interact inside the body. Each question opened a new layer of that map. Each answer helped narrow possibilities and eliminate risks.

Prescribing medication is often imagined as a linear process: identify the problem, choose the drug, write the prescription. In reality, it is far more complex. It resembles problem-solving in motion, where the right choice depends not only on the illness, but on the person experiencing it. Two patients may describe nearly identical symptoms and yet receive different treatments not because one is taken more seriously than the other, but because their bodies, histories, and circumstances are not the same.

The first consideration is always the condition itself. Doctors evaluate what is most likely happening in the body, how the condition typically progresses, and what treatments have been shown to help. But this clinical assessment is only the starting point. From there, the focus widens.

Every medication interacts with the body in specific ways. Doctors must consider how a patient absorbs medication, how it is distributed through tissues, how it is broken down by the liver, and how it is eventually eliminated. These processes are influenced by age, genetics, organ function, and existing medical conditions. A drug that is safe and effective for one person may pose unnecessary risk for another, even when the diagnosis is the same.

Equally important is the broader medical context. Many patients take more than one medication, and drugs do not exist in isolation. They can enhance each other's effects, cancel each other out, or create unwanted side effects when combined. A doctor must consider these interactions carefully. Sometimes, a medication is avoided not because it is ineffective, but because it could complicate an existing treatment plan.

Lifestyle also plays a meaningful role. A medication that causes drowsiness may be unsuitable for someone who drives long distances or operates machinery. A drug that requires strict timing may be difficult for someone with an unpredictable work schedule. Even diet and hydration can influence how a medication behaves. These factors are not peripheral they are central to whether a treatment will succeed outside the clinic.

This is why prescribing often feels slower than patients expect. From the outside, the questions may seem excessive or unrelated. From the clinician's perspective, they are essential safeguards. Each one helps ensure that the treatment fits not just the diagnosis, but the person.

What patients usually encounter is only the final step of this process: the prescription itself. A medication name, a dose, a schedule. The reasoning behind it remains largely unseen. When instructions appear specific or inflexible, it can be tempting to assume they are arbitrary. In reality, they are the distilled outcome of multiple considerations benefits weighed against risks, effectiveness balanced with safety, ideal conditions adjusted to real life.

Medicine is rarely about certainty. It is about choosing the best available option with the information at hand. Doctors work within probabilities, not guarantees. They aim to support the body's natural ability to heal or stabilize while minimizing harm. The prescription represents a decision made at that intersection.

Understanding this does not require blind trust, nor does it demand detailed medical knowledge. It simply invites a shift in perspective. A prescription is not a generic solution applied without thought. It is the result of a careful, individualized process one that considers biology, context, and practicality all at once.

When patients recognize this, medical instructions begin to feel less like rigid rules and more like part of a shared effort. The plan is no longer something imposed from the outside, but something designed with intention. That understanding lays the groundwork for everything that follows.

In the chapters ahead, we will look more closely at how these decisions translate into dosing, timing, and long-term treatment plans. But before moving forward, it is worth holding onto one essential idea: behind every prescription is a process shaped by careful thought, clinical responsibility, and a genuine attempt to treat the person not just the problem.

Chapter 2: The Science of Dosing

When Amina picked up her prescription from the pharmacy, she paused to read the label more carefully than usual. The instructions were precise: one tablet each evening, taken after food, no more and no less. She turned the bottle in her hand, studying its unremarkable appearance. The tablet looked small, almost insignificant. It was difficult to imagine how something so ordinary could require such careful handling.

Her reaction was understandable. Medications are often presented as simple solutions neatly packaged, clearly labeled, and accompanied by brief instructions that seem almost ceremonial. Yet behind those instructions lies one of the most carefully engineered aspects of medical treatment: dosing. Far from being a rough estimate, the dose of a medication represents a deliberate balance between how the body functions and how the drug behaves within it.

At its most basic level, dosing answers a deceptively simple question: how much is enough? But the true answer is rarely straightforward. The human body is dynamic, constantly adjusting to internal and external demands. It absorbs substances, distributes them through tissues, transforms them chemically, and eliminates what it no longer needs. A medication must move through this system without overwhelming it or disappearing before it can be effective.

Doctors consider several factors when determining a dose. One is absorption how much of the medication actually enters the bloodstream. Some drugs are absorbed quickly, others slowly. Some require food to improve absorption, while others are hindered by it. A dose that works well under one condition may be less effective under another, even when the tablet itself is identical.

Another factor is distribution. Once in the bloodstream, a medication does not remain evenly dispersed. It may concentrate in certain tissues, bind to proteins, or cross barriers that protect sensitive organs. These patterns influence both effectiveness and side effects. A dose must be sufficient to reach its target, but not so high that it creates unnecessary strain elsewhere.

Metabolism adds another layer of complexity. Most medications are processed by the liver, where they are chemically altered before being eliminated. The speed of this process varies widely between individuals. Age, genetics, liver function, and other medications all influence how quickly a drug is broken down. A dose that lingers too long may accumulate and cause harm; one that is cleared too quickly may never reach its full effect.

Finally, elimination determines how long a medication remains active. The kidneys play a central role here, filtering substances from the blood and excreting them. If elimination is slowed, even a standard dose can build up over time. If it is accelerated, the medication may need to be given more frequently to maintain its benefit. These considerations are especially important for patients with kidney disease, older adults, and those taking multiple medications.

Because of these variables, dosing is rarely intuitive. It is guided by extensive research, clinical trials, and real-world observation. Patterns emerge when medications are studied across large populations: doses that are consistently effective, ranges that minimize risk, and thresholds beyond which harm becomes more likely. Doctors use this collective knowledge as a foundation, then adjust it to fit the individual sitting in front of them.

This is why taking more medication does not necessarily lead to better results. Beyond a certain point, increasing the dose may offer no additional benefit while increasing the likelihood of side effects. Similarly, reducing a dose without guidance may render a treatment ineffective, even if it feels safer or more conservative. The goal of dosing is not to push the body harder, but to support it precisely.

In everyday life, the science behind dosing remains largely invisible, and that invisibility is intentional. Patients are not expected to calculate absorption rates or metabolic pathways. What matters is recognizing that the dose printed on a label is not arbitrary. It reflects a careful compromise between what the body needs and what it can safely handle.

When people adjust doses on their own taking extra on difficult days or skipping doses when symptoms ease they disrupt that balance. These changes often come from reasonable instincts: a desire for relief, a wish to avoid unnecessary medication, or a belief that the body will regulate itself. Yet even small adjustments can alter how a medication behaves over time, making outcomes less predictable.

Understanding the science of dosing does not require memorization or technical expertise. It requires an appreciation for the fact that each dose represents a thoughtful decision. It is the product of evidence, experience, and caution working together. Doctors aim to provide enough support to make a difference, while preserving the body's ability to adapt and recover.

As we move forward, timing will emerge as another critical dimension of this balance. The amount of medication matters, but so does *when* it enters the body. For now, it is enough to recognize that dosing is not a matter of convenience or habit. It is a deliberate act, designed to align medicine with the body's complex and ever-changing systems.

When patients understand this, the instructions on a label begin to carry new meaning. They are no longer seen as rigid constraints, but as guidance shaped by an intimate understanding of how healing actually works.

Chapter 3: Timing: Why It Matters

When Daniel began his new medication, he approached the instructions with casual flexibility. The label recommended taking it in the morning, but mornings were rarely predictable. Some days he remembered just after lunch, other days late in the evening. The difference seemed trivial. A few hours here or there could not possibly matter, he reasoned. A day was a day, and the body would adjust.

It was only during a follow-up visit that timing entered the conversation. When Daniel mentioned his inconsistent routine, his doctor listened without surprise or disapproval. This was not an unfamiliar story. Daniel had not ignored the instructions; he had simply underestimated their purpose. What felt like a minor detail to him represented an important component of how the medication was designed to work.

The human body does not operate on a flat timeline. Its systems rise and fall in predictable patterns across the day. Hormones fluctuate, digestive activity changes, blood pressure shifts, and the organs responsible for processing medication alter their pace. These rhythms influence how drugs are absorbed, how long they remain active, and how strongly they affect the body at different times.

For this reason, *when* a medication is taken can be as important as *how much* is taken. Some medications work best when the digestive system is active, allowing for smoother absorption. Others are designed to align with periods of rest, supporting processes that occur during sleep. Certain treatments rely on maintaining a steady level in the bloodstream, which requires consistent spacing between doses. Others are meant to act quickly and then fade.

Food adds another layer of complexity. For some medications, taking them with food improves absorption and reduces irritation.

For others, food interferes with how the drug enters the bloodstream. These differences are not intuitive, and they are not visible from the outside. They are the result of how the medication's chemical structure interacts with the body's internal environment.

To patients, these instructions can feel overly precise. "Take in the morning." "Take at night." "Take with food." "Do not take with food." Without context, such guidance may seem rigid or unnecessarily demanding. Yet these details exist because the body responds to patterns. When a medication enters the system in a predictable rhythm, the body adapts. When that rhythm shifts unpredictably, the response becomes less reliable.

Inconsistent timing does not usually cause immediate harm. A single late dose or missed hour rarely undoes progress. The effects are often subtle at first. A medication may seem slightly less effective. Side effects may feel more noticeable. Over time, these small variations can create peaks and dips in drug levels that make treatment outcomes harder to interpret.

This unpredictability affects both patients and clinicians. When a medication does not seem to be working as expected, doctors must consider whether the issue lies with the drug itself, the dose, the condition being treated, or the way the medication is being taken. Inconsistent timing can blur these distinctions, making it difficult to know what adjustments are truly needed.

Consistency, rather than perfection, is the goal. The body does not require exact timing down to the minute, but it does benefit from regularity. When a medication is taken at roughly the same time each day, the body learns what to expect. This allows the treatment to integrate more smoothly into the body's natural rhythms, improving both effectiveness and tolerance.

Life, of course, rarely follows a perfect schedule. Work, travel, family obligations, and unexpected events disrupt routines. These disruptions are not failures; they are part of being human. What matters is awareness. When patients understand *why* timing matters, they are better equipped to make informed choices when routines shift. They can also communicate more clearly with their healthcare providers when consistency becomes difficult.

Timing is not about obedience to a rule. It is about cooperation with the body's internal clock. When medication aligns with that clock, it has a better chance of supporting healing rather than working against natural processes.

As we move into the next chapter, we will explore what happens when treatment plans drift away from their original design not through neglect or defiance, but through ordinary, well-intentioned adjustments. For now, it is enough to remember that time is not just a backdrop to treatment. It is an active participant in how medicine works.

Chapter 4: The Hidden Dangers of Non-Adherence

When Sofia first noticed that her breathing had become easier, relief followed quickly. The tightness in her chest eased, her nights were quieter, and the familiar wheeze that once demanded her attention faded into the background. The inhaler that had occupied a permanent place on her bedside table now spent most of its time forgotten at the bottom of her bag.

One evening, as she prepared for sleep, she hesitated with the inhaler in her hand. She felt well better than she had in months. Taking it seemed unnecessary. So she skipped it. Nothing happened. The next night, she skipped it again. Days passed, then weeks. The absence of symptoms felt like confirmation that she no longer needed the medication.

What Sofia experienced is one of the most common turning points in long-term treatment: improvement mistaken for resolution. When symptoms fade, it is natural to assume the problem has disappeared. In many cases, however, the improvement is not evidence that the condition is gone it is evidence that the treatment is working. When the treatment is withdrawn, the underlying condition often returns, quietly at first, then more noticeably.

Non-adherence, the term used when treatment plans are not followed as intended, is often misunderstood. It is rarely a matter of carelessness or defiance. More often, it arises from reasonable human impulses: the desire to feel normal again, the wish to reduce dependence on medication, or the simple need to simplify daily routines. These motivations are understandable, and they deserve empathy. Yet they can carry consequences that are not immediately apparent.

Some medications depend on consistency to maintain their effect. When doses are skipped or taken irregularly, drug levels in the body fluctuate. These fluctuations can reduce effectiveness or increase side effects, even when the total amount taken over time seems similar. The body responds to patterns, and when those patterns change, the response changes with them.

In other cases, stopping treatment too early allows a condition to regain momentum. Symptoms may return gradually, making it difficult to connect the relapse to earlier decisions. By the time the connection becomes clear, the condition may be more difficult to control than it was initially. This progression can feel confusing and discouraging, especially when the patient believed they were improving.

There are also situations in which non-adherence affects more than the individual. Treatments designed to manage infectious diseases, for example, often rely on completing a full course. When treatment is interrupted, it can influence how the illness behaves, both in the individual and, in some cases, within the broader community. These effects are rarely visible at the personal level, but they are part of the larger context clinicians consider when prescribing.

None of this is meant to imply that patients must follow instructions without question. Medical care is not about rigid compliance; it is about informed participation. Life is unpredictable, and perfect adherence is rarely realistic. What matters is understanding why a plan exists and what may happen when it changes.

When patients see instructions as arbitrary rules, deviations feel harmless. When they understand the purpose behind those instructions, they are more likely to recognize when a change carries risk. This understanding also encourages communication. Instead of silently adjusting a plan, patients who understand its logic are more likely to ask questions, express concerns, and seek guidance when something feels unsustainable.

The dangers of non-adherence are often hidden not because they are dramatic, but because they unfold quietly. They appear as subtle shifts rather than sudden events. They develop over time rather than all at once. Recognizing this helps reframe treatment as an ongoing process rather than a temporary task.

For Sofia, the return of her symptoms was not a failure. It was a lesson. When she spoke with her doctor, she learned that the inhaler was not just a response to symptoms, but a tool designed to prevent them. With that understanding, her relationship with the medication changed. It no longer felt like an unnecessary obligation, but like a form of maintenance quiet, protective, and purposeful.

As we move into the next chapter, we will look more closely at the psychological forces that shape adherence. Why good intentions fade. Why routines unravel. And why understanding alone is sometimes not enough. Before turning the page, it is worth holding onto one central idea: treatment does not work only when symptoms are present. Often, it works precisely because it prevents them from returning.

Chapter 5: The Psychology of Following Instructions

When Malik was first told he had high blood pressure, he responded with resolve. He listened carefully as his doctor explained the treatment plan, asked questions, and left the clinic determined to do everything correctly. At home, he set reminders on his phone, arranged his medications neatly on the kitchen counter, and followed the instructions with careful attention. For a while, the routine felt manageable, even reassuring. It gave him a sense of control.

Then life intervened.

A late night turned into a rushed morning. A long workday blurred into an evening of fatigue. A weekend trip disrupted his carefully built habits. None of these moments felt significant on their own. He still cared about his health. He still believed the treatment mattered. Yet the structure he had created began to loosen, not suddenly, but gradually.

Malik's experience reflects a quiet reality of medical care: adherence is not determined by knowledge alone. People can understand instructions clearly and still struggle to follow them consistently. This gap is not a failure of character or discipline. It is the result of how human behavior actually works.

One of the strongest psychological influences is perception. When symptoms improve, people often conclude that the problem has resolved. When symptoms persist, they may question whether the treatment is effective at all. Both responses are logical from a human standpoint. Improvement brings relief and a desire to return to normal life. Persistence brings frustration and doubt. In either case, the treatment plan becomes vulnerable to adjustment.

Another powerful force is habit. Medical instructions often require behaviors that did not previously exist taking medication at a specific time, avoiding certain foods, monitoring bodily changes. These actions must be repeated consistently before they become automatic. When routines are disrupted, even briefly, restarting them can feel surprisingly difficult. The mind gravitates toward what is familiar and effortless, especially under stress.

Emotion also plays a significant role. Fear of side effects, concern about long-term dependence, or discomfort with the idea of "needing" medication can influence behavior in subtle ways. These feelings may never be spoken aloud. Instead, they surface as small decisions delaying a dose, taking less than prescribed, or skipping treatment altogether. These choices are not acts of rebellion. They are attempts to regain control in situations that feel uncertain.

There is also the influence of mental load. Managing health often becomes one responsibility among many. Work, family, finances, and personal obligations compete for attention. When cognitive resources are stretched thin, even well-intentioned routines can fall apart. Forgetting a dose is rarely a conscious decision; it is often the result of exhaustion or distraction.

Communication gaps further complicate adherence. When instructions feel overwhelming or unclear, people fill in the gaps with assumptions. When questions go unasked, misunderstandings persist. Many patients hesitate to admit confusion or difficulty, believing they should already know how to manage their care. In reality, confusion is not a weakness it is a signal that more explanation is needed.

What emerges from all of this is a simple truth: following medical instructions is not just a medical task. It is a psychological process shaped by emotion, habit, perception, and circumstance. Willpower alone is rarely enough. Understanding the human side of adherence helps explain why even motivated, intelligent people struggle at times.

This understanding shifts the conversation away from blame and toward compassion. Instead of asking why someone failed to follow instructions, it becomes more useful to ask what made adherence difficult. Was the routine unrealistic? Were fears unaddressed? Was the explanation incomplete? These questions open the door to solutions that are both medically sound and realistically sustainable.

For Malik, the turning point came not from stricter reminders, but from an honest conversation. When he admitted to his doctor that he had struggled to maintain the routine, he was met not with disappointment, but with understanding. Together, they adjusted the plan to better fit his daily life. The treatment did not change dramatically, but his ability to follow it did.

The psychology of adherence reminds us that treatment plans do not exist in isolation. They live within the complexities of real lives. When patients understand their own behavioral patterns and feel supported in discussing them, adherence becomes less about obligation and more about alignment.

In the next chapter, we will explore how communication between patients and clinicians can bridge the gap between intention and action. Before moving forward, it is worth remembering this: struggling to follow instructions does not mean you do not care about your health. It means you are human. And healthcare works best when it is designed with that humanity in mind.

Chapter 6: How to Talk to Your Doctor

Laila arrived for her appointment with a clear intention. Over the past week, she had noticed new symptoms and written down questions in a small notebook, determined not to forget them. Yet as she sat in the examination room and the conversation began, that resolve quietly dissolved. The doctor spoke efficiently, the visit felt brief, and before she realized it, the appointment was over. She left with answers to questions she hadn't asked and instructions she only partially understood.

That evening, as she opened her notebook again, the questions were still there unanswered.

Laila's experience is not unusual. Many patients find it surprisingly difficult to speak openly with their doctors, even when they care deeply about their health. Time pressure, unfamiliar terminology, and the inherent imbalance of expertise can make conversations feel one-sided. Patients may worry about sounding uninformed, taking too much time, or appearing confrontational. As a result, uncertainty often goes unspoken.

Yet communication is one of the most powerful tools in medical care. Doctors rely on what patients share to make informed decisions, and patients rely on doctors to explain those decisions clearly. When communication falters, gaps form small at first, but capable of shaping outcomes in meaningful ways. Instructions may be misunderstood, concerns left unaddressed, and assumptions quietly substituted for clarity.

Talking to a doctor is not about challenging authority or mastering medical language. It is about participating in a shared process. Doctors bring scientific training, clinical experience, and a broad understanding of disease. Patients bring lived experience the details of their symptoms, routines, fears, and priorities. Effective care depends on both perspectives being present.

One of the most important shifts patients can make is recognizing that questions are not interruptions. They are an essential part of the conversation. When something is unclear, asking for clarification is not a sign of ignorance; it is a sign of engagement. Simple questions *What does this medication do? Why is the timing important? What should I expect?* can transform confusion into understanding.

Honesty is equally important. Patients sometimes adjust their treatment routines without mentioning it, not out of deception, but out of embarrassment or fear of being judged. Yet these details matter. When doctors understand what is actually happening outside the clinic, they can explain the reasoning behind a plan more clearly or adapt it to better fit the patient's reality. Open communication creates space for practical solutions rather than silent struggle.

It is also worth acknowledging that doctors are human. They work within time constraints, manage complex caseloads, and make decisions under pressure. This does not diminish their commitment, but it means that communication works best when both sides participate actively. A brief pause to gather thoughts, a request for clarification, or a statement such as *I'm not sure I understand this yet* can redirect the conversation toward clarity.

Patients do not need to become experts in medicine. Their role is not to diagnose or prescribe, but to articulate their experience as accurately as possible. Describing how symptoms feel, when they occur, what interferes with daily life, and what feels manageable provides clinicians with critical information. When patients speak openly about their concerns and constraints, treatment plans become more realistic and effective.

This kind of communication also builds trust. When patients feel heard, they are more likely to follow treatment plans and to raise concerns early. When doctors understand their patients' realities, they can offer guidance that feels supportive rather than prescriptive. Over time, this exchange strengthens the partnership at the heart of healthcare.

As we move into the next chapter, we will see how these principles play out through real-world scenarios fictional stories that reflect common challenges in understanding and following treatment plans. Before turning the page, it is worth holding onto one essential idea: talking to your doctor is not a test of knowledge or confidence. It is a conversation. And like any meaningful conversation, it works best when both sides speak honestly, listen carefully, and share responsibility for understanding.

Part II: Where Understanding Breaks Down

Common Misinterpretations and the Logic Behind Them

Medical misunderstandings rarely come from ignorance. More often, they emerge from logic applied without context. Patients observe how they feel, draw conclusions that make sense in daily life, and adjust their behavior accordingly. These conclusions are not careless; they are reasonable attempts to regain control in situations filled with uncertainty.

The problem is not that patients think incorrectly. It is that they think incompletely without access to the full framework clinicians use when designing treatment plans. When that framework is missing, even intelligent, well-intentioned reasoning can lead to decisions that quietly undermine care.

This section examines some of the most common interpretations patients make when navigating treatment. Each chapter focuses on one belief that feels intuitive, one fictional case that brings it to life, and one clinical explanation that reframes the logic behind it. The goal is not correction through instruction, but understanding through perspective.

Chapter 7: "If I Feel Better, I Can Stop"

When Nadia first noticed that her symptoms were fading, relief washed over her quickly. The discomfort that had dominated her days was finally easing. Her energy was returning, her sleep improving, and the constant reminder that something was wrong had softened into the background. For the first time since starting treatment, she felt like herself again.

That was when the question surfaced.

One evening, as she prepared to take her medication, she paused. The bottle felt heavier than usual in her hand not physically, but symbolically. She no longer felt sick. Continuing treatment began to feel unnecessary, even excessive. After all, she reasoned, the purpose of the medication was to make her feel better. And she did feel better.

So she skipped a dose.

Nothing happened. The next day felt just as good. Encouraged by the absence of consequences, she skipped another. Within a week, she had quietly stopped altogether. She didn't see herself as abandoning treatment; she saw herself as responding to evidence. Her body felt fine. The problem, in her mind, had resolved.

This conclusion is one of the most common and most understandable misinterpretations in medical care. In everyday life, improvement usually signals completion. When pain subsides, we stop resting the injury. When a task is finished, we put the tools away. It feels logical to apply the same reasoning to treatment.

But medicine often operates on a different timeline.

In many conditions, symptoms are not the disease itself. They are signals surface indicators of an underlying process. Treatment may suppress those signals without eliminating the condition that caused them. When the treatment stops, the process continues quietly until it reaches a point where symptoms return.

From a clinical perspective, Nadia's improvement was not a signal to stop. It was evidence that the treatment was doing exactly what it was designed to do.

Doctors often prescribe medication not only to relieve symptoms, but to stabilize systems, prevent recurrence, or interrupt a process that would otherwise persist. In these cases, the absence of symptoms does not mean the job is finished. It means the system is being held in balance.

This distinction is rarely obvious to patients because it runs counter to everyday experience. Feeling better feels like proof. And without explanation, that proof is persuasive.

The danger lies in what happens next. When treatment stops prematurely, the underlying condition often resumes its course. But it rarely does so dramatically. Symptoms may return slowly, subtly, or inconsistently. When they do, patients are often confused. The medication worked once why did it fail now?

In reality, it didn't fail. It was removed too soon.

This pattern can be emotionally frustrating. Patients may feel discouraged, mistrustful, or reluctant to restart treatment. Some interpret the relapse as evidence that their condition is worsening or that the medication is ineffective. The original logic I felt better, so I stopped is replaced by a second misunderstanding it didn't really work after all.

Reframing this belief requires shifting how improvement is interpreted.

Feeling better does not always mean the condition is gone. Often, it means the treatment is actively maintaining balance. The goal of care is not always immediate relief; sometimes it is prevention, stabilization, or protection against future harm. In these cases, continuation is not redundancy it is function.

This does not mean patients should never stop treatment. It means stopping should be a decision, not a reaction. When improvement triggers questions, those questions deserve conversation rather than silence. A brief discussion can clarify whether symptoms are a signal of resolution or a response being maintained.

When patients understand this distinction, treatment changes character. It no longer feels like an obligation extended beyond necessity. It becomes a strategy with a purpose one that may continue even when symptoms fade.

Improvement is meaningful. It should be welcomed. But in medicine, improvement is sometimes a milestone not the finish line.

Chapter 8: "If I Feel Worse, It's Not Working"

When Marcus began his new treatment, he approached it with cautious optimism. He had read the information sheet carefully, noted the possible side effects, and prepared himself for mild discomfort. What he didn't expect was how quickly his body would react. Within days, he felt more fatigued than usual. His appetite dipped. A low, persistent unease settled into his routine.

Instead of improvement, he felt worse.

By the end of the first week, doubt had replaced optimism. The conclusion felt unavoidable: the medication was not working. In fact, it seemed to be doing the opposite. Why would a treatment designed to help make him feel worse? The logic was simple and emotionally compelling. If the problem was being treated correctly, symptoms should improve not intensify.

So Marcus began to disengage. He skipped doses on days he felt particularly uncomfortable. He considered stopping altogether. The worsening symptoms felt like evidence, and evidence, in everyday reasoning, demands response.

This interpretation is one of the most common turning points in treatment. It arises from a deeply ingrained expectation: that improvement should be immediate and linear. In most areas of life, effort produces visible results. Pain relief, task completion, recovery all tend to move in one direction. Medicine, however, often does not follow that pattern.

From a clinical perspective, early discomfort does not necessarily indicate failure. In many treatments, the initial phase involves adjustment. The body is responding to a new influence, recalibrating systems that may have been operating under strain for a long time. This adjustment period can bring temporary discomfort before stability is achieved.

Some medications require time to reach effective levels in the body. Others initiate processes that unfold gradually. In these cases, early symptoms do not reflect the final outcome. They reflect transition.

This concept is difficult to grasp without explanation because it conflicts with instinct. Feeling worse feels like harm. And without context, patients are left to interpret that sensation on their own.

Clinicians understand that timing matters not just when medication is taken, but when its benefits are expected to emerge. They anticipate that some treatments may initially feel uncomfortable before improvement becomes apparent. This is why follow-up timelines are often specified. Improvement is assessed not immediately, but over weeks rather than days.

When this context is missing, patients may draw conclusions prematurely. A treatment that requires patience is abandoned before it has the opportunity to help. When that happens, the medication is labeled ineffective, even though it was never given the conditions it required to succeed.

There is also a psychological layer to this misinterpretation. Starting treatment often heightens attention to bodily sensations. People notice changes more acutely, monitoring themselves for signs of improvement or harm. This increased awareness can amplify discomfort that might otherwise pass unnoticed. The body feels different, and difference is easily interpreted as danger.

The result is a feedback loop. Discomfort fuels anxiety. Anxiety sharpens perception. Sharpened perception magnifies discomfort. In this loop, the treatment becomes associated with harm, even when the underlying process is benign or temporary.

Reframing this belief requires a shift in expectations.

Feeling worse does not automatically mean something is wrong. It may mean the body is adapting. The key distinction is between expected adjustment and true harm. That distinction cannot always be made in isolation. It requires guidance.

This is why communication matters so deeply during the early stages of treatment. When patients know what to expect how long adjustment may last, which symptoms are typical, and which are not uncertainty loses some of its power. Discomfort becomes information rather than alarm.

This does not mean patients should ignore worsening symptoms. It means they should interpret them within a framework rather than in isolation. When discomfort is unexpected, severe, or progressive, it warrants attention. But when it aligns with known patterns of adjustment, it may simply require time.

Marcus eventually spoke with his clinician, expecting to hear that the medication was unsuitable. Instead, he learned that the timeline he was using to judge effectiveness was misaligned with how the treatment worked. With that understanding, his experience shifted. The discomfort no longer felt like evidence of failure. It felt like a phase with an endpoint.

Within weeks, improvement followed.

The misconception that "feeling worse means it isn't working" arises because it relies on everyday logic applied to an unfamiliar system. Once the system is explained, the logic changes. Treatment is no longer judged by immediate comfort, but by trajectory.

Early discomfort is not always a sign to stop. Sometimes, it is a sign to understand.

Chapter 9: "Lower Dose = Safer"

When Elena adjusted her medication, she did so quietly and with what felt like careful reasoning. The prescribed dose seemed strong, perhaps more than she truly needed. She worried about long-term effects, about burdening her body unnecessarily. So she decided to take a little less cutting tablets in half, spacing doses farther apart, convincing herself that moderation was the responsible choice.

She didn't stop treatment. She refined it.

At first, the change felt reassuring. Taking a lower dose gave her a sense of control and safety. If medication carried risk, then less of it must carry less risk. The logic felt sound, almost self-evident. In everyday life, moderation is usually wise. Smaller portions, lighter exertion, gentler force less is often safer.

But in medicine, this assumption can be misleading.

From a clinical standpoint, a prescribed dose is not a maximum tolerated limit. It is a target a level chosen because it reliably produces a desired effect within a defined safety margin. Doses are not selected to push the body to its edge; they are chosen to sit within a therapeutic window, where benefit outweighs risk.

Below that window, the medication may no longer do what it was intended to do.

Many treatments require a minimum effective dose to influence the body in a meaningful way. Below that threshold, the drug may circulate without achieving its purpose. The patient remains exposed to the medication, but without gaining its benefit. In this situation, "less" is not safer it is simply ineffective.

This distinction is difficult to appreciate because it runs counter to intuition. Risk is often imagined as linear: more exposure equals more danger. In reality, medical risk is contextual. A medication that is ineffective does not become harmless simply because the dose is lower. It may still interact with the body, still require processing by the liver and kidneys, still carry side effects while failing to deliver its intended support.

There is also a hidden cost to underdosing. When a treatment appears ineffective, patients and clinicians may conclude that the medication itself is unsuitable. The dose is not questioned; the drug is. This can lead to unnecessary changes, escalation to more complex treatments, or abandonment of an approach that might have worked if used as designed.

In some conditions, underdosing carries additional consequences. In treatments where consistency and adequate exposure are essential, insufficient dosing can allow a condition to persist in a weakened but unresolved state. This partial suppression can complicate future treatment, making the condition harder to manage over time.

Elena's experience reflected this pattern. After weeks of taking a reduced dose, she felt little improvement. Her symptoms lingered, sometimes improving slightly, sometimes returning. The inconsistency reinforced her belief that the medication was not right for her. When she finally discussed her routine with her clinician, the issue became clear not as a reprimand, but as an explanation.

The prescribed dose had been chosen to reach a specific effect. By staying below it, she had remained just outside the range where improvement could occur.

Reframing this misconception requires a shift in how safety is understood.

Safety in medicine is not achieved by minimizing exposure at all costs. It is achieved by balancing exposure with purpose. A dose that is too high can cause harm, but a dose that is too low can also fail to protect. Both fall outside the intended therapeutic window.

This does not mean that dosing should never be adjusted. It means adjustments should be guided, not assumed. When patients feel uncomfortable with a prescribed dose, that discomfort is a signal for conversation not self-correction. Clinicians can often explain why a dose was chosen, adjust it safely if needed, or offer alternatives that align better with a patient's concerns.

Once Elena understood this framework, the prescription no longer felt excessive. It felt intentional. Taking the full dose became less about risk and more about alignment trusting the balance that had been carefully considered.

"Lower dose equals safer" feels responsible because it borrows logic from everyday life. But medicine operates within narrower margins. In that space, effectiveness and safety are not opposites. They are partners.

Chapter 10: Natural Means Harmless

When Sara decided to stop her prescribed medication, she did not feel reckless. She felt careful. The new regimen she chose felt gentler, more aligned with her values. The supplements were labeled natural. The ingredients were familiar, drawn from plants rather than laboratories. Friends spoke highly of them. Online testimonials described healing without side effects. Compared to the clinical language of prescription drugs, this approach felt safer almost intuitive.

Natural, she believed, meant harmless.

For a time, the decision brought comfort. Taking the supplements felt empowering. They fit easily into her routine and carried none of the anxiety she associated with medication warnings and long lists of potential side effects. The absence of immediate discomfort reinforced her confidence. Her body, she assumed, would respond better to something derived from nature.

This belief is deeply ingrained, and it is not unreasonable. In everyday life, natural often signals familiarity and safety. We associate it with food, with tradition, with things the body has encountered before. Artificial, by contrast, suggests intrusion something foreign and potentially dangerous. It is natural to extend this logic to healthcare.

But medicine does not divide neatly along these lines.

From a clinical perspective, "natural" describes origin, not effect. A substance's source does not determine how it behaves in the body. Many of the most powerful medicines in use today originated from plants. Many naturally occurring substances are capable of significant harm. Nature produces remedies and poisons with equal ease.

What matters in treatment is not whether something is natural or synthetic, but how it interacts with the body. Does it alter physiology? Does it affect organs? Does it interact with other substances? These questions apply equally to prescription medications, supplements, and herbal products.

One of the risks associated with the "natural equals harmless" belief is that it lowers vigilance. People are less likely to scrutinize doses, interactions, or side effects when a product feels familiar or benign. Supplements are often taken without the same caution applied to prescription drugs, even though they can influence the body in meaningful ways.

Another complication lies in regulation. Prescription medications undergo extensive testing to establish dosing, effectiveness, and safety. Supplements and herbal products often do not face the same level of scrutiny. This does not mean they are ineffective or dangerous by default, but it does mean that their effects may be less predictable. Dosage can vary between products, and interactions may be poorly documented.

Sara encountered this unpredictability gradually. After several weeks, she noticed subtle changes unusual fatigue, digestive discomfort, fluctuations in how she felt day to day. Because she did not associate supplements with risk, she did not immediately consider them as a cause. When her symptoms worsened, she assumed her original condition was progressing rather than questioning her new regimen.

It was only after a detailed conversation with her clinician that the connection emerged. The supplements she was taking interacted with other treatments she had not fully discontinued. The combination altered how her body processed both. Nothing about the situation was dramatic or malicious. It was simply unexamined.

Reframing this misconception requires separating comfort from safety.

Familiar language can be reassuring, but it is not a substitute for understanding. Natural substances can be beneficial, neutral, or harmful depending on context, dose, and interaction. They deserve the same thoughtful consideration as any other treatment.

This does not mean rejecting non-prescription approaches or dismissing alternative therapies. It means integrating them consciously. When patients share what they are taking whether prescribed, purchased, or recommended by others clinicians can assess the full picture. Transparency restores balance.

For Sara, acknowledging that "natural" did not mean "risk-free" changed how she approached her care. She did not abandon her preference for gentler options, but she learned to evaluate them with the same seriousness she applied to medication. The shift was subtle but important. It replaced assumption with inquiry.

Nature offers powerful tools. Medicine does as well. Safety emerges not from origin, but from understanding.

Chapter 11: Side Effects Mean Damage

When Thomas noticed the tremor in his hands, panic followed quickly. It was subtle at first barely visible unless he paid close attention. But once he noticed it, he couldn't unsee it. The timing felt unmistakable. He had started a new medication just weeks earlier. The conclusion formed immediately: the drug was harming him.

He searched the information leaflet again, scanning the list of possible side effects. There it was tremor, listed among others. Seeing it in print did not reassure him. It confirmed his fear. Side effects, in his mind, were evidence of damage. Something was going wrong inside his body, and the medication was the cause.

That night, he skipped his dose.

This belief that side effects indicate harm is one of the most emotionally charged misinterpretations in treatment. Unlike other misconceptions, it is driven not just by logic, but by fear. The body feels different, sometimes uncomfortable, sometimes alarming. When that sensation is linked to a medication, the instinct to stop feels protective, even urgent.

In everyday life, discomfort often signals injury. Pain tells us to withdraw our hand from a hot surface. Nausea warns us that something may be wrong. It makes sense to apply the same reasoning to treatment. If a medication causes unpleasant sensations, it must be damaging the body.

In medicine, however, side effects do not all mean harm.

From a clinical perspective, a side effect is simply an effect that is not the primary therapeutic goal. It may be benign, transient, or an expected consequence of how the medication works. Many treatments influence systems that extend beyond their intended target. As the body adapts, these effects often diminish or resolve entirely.

The challenge lies in distinguishing between expected side effects and true adverse reactions. Expected side effects are known, studied, and anticipated. They are part of the risk–benefit balance that informs prescribing decisions. Adverse reactions, by contrast, signal genuine harm and require prompt action. Without context, patients are left to interpret both through sensation alone.

This distinction is rarely intuitive. Feeling uncomfortable feels dangerous, regardless of cause. And when patients lack a framework for interpreting these sensations, fear fills the gap.

Thomas's tremor, while unsettling, fell into the category of an expected and usually temporary effect. It reflected how the medication interacted with his nervous system as his body adjusted. With time, it would likely diminish. But Thomas did not know this. Without explanation, the symptom became a threat rather than a signal.

Another complicating factor is attention. Starting a new treatment often heightens awareness of bodily changes. Sensations that might previously have gone unnoticed become magnified. This increased vigilance can amplify normal fluctuations, making them feel abnormal or alarming.

The result is a cascade. Sensation leads to fear. Fear leads to avoidance. Avoidance leads to inconsistent treatment. And inconsistency makes it harder to determine whether symptoms are improving, worsening, or unrelated.

Reframing this misconception requires redefining what side effects represent.

Side effects are not automatically signs of damage. They are information. They indicate how the body is responding to an intervention. Some responses are acceptable and temporary. Others are not. The difference lies not in how uncomfortable the sensation feels, but in what it signifies physiologically.

This is why communication is critical when starting treatment. When patients know which effects are expected, which are temporary, and which require immediate attention, fear loses its urgency. Sensations become data points rather than alarms.

This does not mean patients should ignore side effects or endure distress silently. It means they should interpret sensations within a framework rather than in isolation. Reporting side effects allows clinicians to adjust treatment, provide reassurance, or intervene when necessary. Silence, by contrast, leaves patients alone with uncertainty.

When Thomas finally spoke with his clinician, the explanation changed his response entirely. The tremor was addressed, monitored, and contextualized. It did not disappear overnight, but it lost its power. Understanding replaced fear, and consistency replaced avoidance.

The belief that "side effects mean damage" persists because it draws from everyday survival instincts. But medicine often requires a more nuanced interpretation. Not every signal indicates danger. Some indicate transition.

Learning to tell the difference does not require medical expertise. It requires conversation.

Closing the Section

The misconceptions explored in this section share a common origin. They arise when reasonable human logic is applied without clinical context. Feeling better suggests stopping. Feeling worse suggests failure. Less feels safer. Natural feels gentle. Discomfort feels dangerous.

None of these conclusions are foolish. They are incomplete.

When the reasoning behind treatment is understood, these interpretations lose their grip. Decisions become informed rather than reactive. Treatment becomes a collaboration rather than a guessing game.

With this foundation, we now return to the broader picture how understanding, communication, and partnership shape long-term care and patient education in an increasingly complex healthcare world.

PART III Integration, Education, and the Future of Partnership

By this point, the mechanics of misunderstanding are no longer abstract. The previous section did not present errors to be corrected, but patterns to be recognized ways reasonable people interpret their experiences when information is incomplete or context is missing. These interpretations did not arise from indifference or carelessness. They emerged from logic applied in isolation.

Understanding where reasoning breaks down is necessary, but it is not sufficient.

Healthcare does not occur in controlled environments. It unfolds over time, within real lives shaped by work, family, fatigue, fear, and hope. Decisions are not made once and followed indefinitely; they are revisited, adjusted, questioned, and sometimes abandoned. In this landscape, understanding must do more than inform it must endure.

This final section shifts focus from individual misconceptions to the broader system in which they arise. It asks how understanding is reinforced, how communication evolves, and how education must adapt to support patients beyond the moment instructions are given. It recognizes that clarity is not a single achievement, but an ongoing process.

The chapters that follow bring the book's ideas back together. They show how misunderstanding accumulates quietly across time, how explanation can restore alignment, and how partnership not authority alone sustains care. They also look forward, examining how patient education must change in a healthcare environment defined by information abundance and increasing complexity.

This section does not offer solutions in the form of rules or strategies. Instead, it offers a framework for thinking one that acknowledges uncertainty, respects human behavior, and treats understanding as a shared responsibility.

If the earlier parts of this book explained how medical decisions are made and why they are misunderstood, this final section explores what happens next: how understanding is maintained, how it fails, and how it can be strengthened in a system that depends on trust.

Healthcare does not succeed through precision alone. It succeeds through alignment between explanation and experience, intention and action, knowledge and life. What follows is not a conclusion, but a convergence.

Chapter 12: Case-Based Integration: How Misunderstanding Quietly Shapes Care

By the time patients reach this point in their healthcare journey, they rarely lack information. They have heard explanations, read labels, followed instructions, and made sincere efforts to do the right thing. And yet, as the previous chapters have shown, misunderstanding still finds its way in not through negligence, but through logic applied without context.

This chapter does not introduce new misconceptions. Instead, it shows how several of them often coexist, overlap, and reinforce one another in real life. Rarely does a patient struggle with only one mistaken belief. More often, treatment drifts because multiple small interpretations accumulate quietly over time.

Consider Priya.

On the surface, her routine looked responsible. She took her medication daily, organized her pills carefully, and rarely missed a dose. From the outside, nothing appeared wrong. Yet over time, subtle discomforts began to surface fatigue, occasional dizziness, a vague sense that something was off. She could not point to a single cause, and so she adjusted what felt reasonable.

She shifted timing to suit her schedule. She reduced doses on days she felt well. When she felt worse, she questioned whether the medication was helping at all. Each decision made sense on its own. Together, they gradually moved her treatment further from its original design.

Priya did not see herself as non-adherent. She saw herself as thoughtful.

When she finally described her routine in detail, the pattern became clear. Her experience reflected not one misunderstanding, but several: improvement mistaken for resolution, flexibility mistaken for harmlessness, discomfort mistaken for failure. None of these beliefs were reckless. They were incomplete.

Another example comes from Jonas, whose challenge was less about logic and more about silence. He valued independence and believed that managing treatment should be straightforward. When his routine became inconsistent, he did not mention it. Missing doses felt like a personal shortcoming, not a clinical issue worth discussing.

Over time, his symptoms fluctuated unpredictably. Some days were stable, others exhausting. Because the pattern did not match his expectations, he attributed it to stress or aging. The possibility that his routine played a role never fully surfaced not because he didn't care, but because he assumed he should already be handling it.

Jonas's case illustrates how misunderstanding is often reinforced by isolation. Without conversation, assumptions go unchallenged. Treatment becomes something to manage privately rather than collaboratively. When he finally spoke openly, the relief came not from a dramatic change in medication, but from shared understanding.

Hana's story adds another layer. Her struggle was shaped by fear. Side effects unsettled her, and uncertainty made consistency difficult. She delayed doses, skipped others, and monitored her body closely for signs of harm. The irregularity made it impossible to distinguish between side effects, anxiety, and the underlying condition itself.

In her case, misunderstanding was not about belief, but interpretation. Sensation became threat. Discomfort became damage. Without a framework to interpret what she felt, every signal carried weight.

What these cases reveal is not patient failure, but a predictable pattern. When understanding is partial, patients compensate by reasoning the best way they know how. They observe, interpret, and adjust. The problem is not that they think they think constantly. The problem is that they are often thinking alone.

Clinicians, by contrast, operate within a broader framework. They understand timelines, thresholds, adaptation phases, and trade-offs. When that framework is not shared, patients are left to bridge the gap themselves. The result is not chaos, but quiet drift.

This is why education and communication cannot be isolated events. A single explanation at the beginning of treatment is rarely sufficient. Understanding evolves as experience evolves. Questions arise not at the moment instructions are given, but weeks later, when real life collides with theory.

Case-based integration matters because it mirrors how healthcare unfolds. People do not encounter misconceptions in neat categories. They encounter them in lived moments when they feel better, when they feel worse, when something feels uncomfortable, when something feels unnecessary. Each moment invites interpretation.

When patients have access to the reasoning behind treatment, these moments become opportunities for dialogue rather than decision points made in isolation. Treatment plans remain flexible without becoming fragile. Adjustments become collaborative rather than reactive.

This chapter sits where it does for a reason. After exploring where understanding breaks down, it brings the pieces back together. It shows that adherence is not about discipline, intelligence, or intention. It is about alignment between expectation and reality, between explanation and experience.

As we move forward to the future of patient education, one truth stands out clearly: understanding is not delivered once and retained forever. It is built, tested, revised, and reinforced over time. When that process is supported, care becomes not only more effective, but more humane.

Chapter 13: The Future of Patient Education

When Omar returned home from his appointment, he did what many patients do when uncertainty lingers: he searched for answers online. Within minutes, he found an overwhelming mix of articles, videos, forums, and personal stories. Some sources contradicted others. Some amplified fear. Others offered reassurance without evidence. The more he read, the less confident he felt. He closed his laptop with the uneasy sense that access to information had not translated into understanding.

Omar's experience reflects a defining challenge of modern healthcare. Patients today are surrounded by information, yet clarity often remains elusive. The future of patient education is not about providing more facts. It is about helping people interpret, evaluate, and apply information in ways that support real decisions in real lives.

For much of medical history, education flowed in one direction. Clinicians spoke, patients listened, and instructions were expected to be followed. That model is no longer sufficient. As patients take a more active role in their care, education must shift from instruction to explanation. Understanding becomes the goal, not compliance.

This shift requires a deeper emphasis on communication. Healthcare professionals are increasingly recognizing that effective education depends on how information is delivered, not just what is delivered. Explanations must meet patients where they are accounting for their level of health literacy, cultural background, emotional state, and daily constraints. Clarity is not simplification; it is precision expressed in accessible language.

Technology is reshaping this landscape in meaningful ways. Patient portals, telehealth visits, medication reminders, and digital education platforms now extend care beyond the clinic. These tools allow patients to revisit instructions, track progress, and communicate questions more easily. When used thoughtfully, they reduce the burden of remembering and lower the barrier to asking for help.

Yet technology alone cannot resolve the deeper challenge Omar faced. Algorithms do not replace judgment, and access does not guarantee understanding. Without context, even accurate information can mislead. The future of patient education depends on curation guiding patients toward reliable sources and helping them interpret what they find.

Storytelling plays a crucial role here. Humans do not learn through data alone; they learn through narratives that reflect experience. When medical concepts are embedded in relatable stories, they become easier to understand and remember. Stories give shape to abstract ideas and show how decisions unfold over time. They do not replace science, but they translate it into lived reality.

Another essential element of the future is inclusivity. Patients differ widely in language, culture, beliefs, and access to care. Educational approaches that assume a single perspective inevitably leave many people behind. Effective patient education must acknowledge these differences and adapt accordingly. This is not merely a logistical concern it is an ethical one. Understanding should not be a privilege reserved for those fluent in medical language.

Transparency also matters. Medicine continues to evolve, and uncertainty is an inherent part of that evolution. When clinicians acknowledge what is known, what is uncertain, and what is still being studied, patients gain a more realistic understanding of their care. This openness builds trust and reduces the anxiety that often arises when expectations are misaligned with reality.

For patients, the future of education means greater partnership. It means being able to ask questions without hesitation, to access information without being overwhelmed, and to understand treatment plans well enough to engage with them meaningfully. Education becomes less about memorizing instructions and more about developing confidence.

For clinicians, it means embracing education as an ongoing process rather than a one-time explanation. Understanding grows through repetition, dialogue, and reflection. When patients are supported in this way, adherence improves not because they are told what to do, but because they understand why it matters.

As we move into the final chapter, one theme stands out clearly. Patient education is not an add-on to medical care; it is a foundation of it. When understanding is prioritized, confusion loses its grip, and partnership becomes possible. In a healthcare system that grows more complex each year, clarity is not a luxury. It is a necessity.

Chapter 14: Conclusion: Your Health Is a Partnership

When Elena stepped out of her doctor's office that afternoon, nothing about her treatment plan had changed. The medication was the same. The schedule was the same. The condition itself remained. What had changed was something less visible but far more important her understanding. For the first time, the instructions she had been following felt connected to a larger logic. They no longer read as isolated rules, but as part of a conversation she now felt included in.

Elena's experience reflects the central message of this book. Healthcare is often framed as a series of directives: diagnoses given, prescriptions written, instructions handed over. But beneath those transactions lies a relationship. When that relationship is built on understanding rather than assumption, treatment becomes more than a task to complete. It becomes a shared effort.

Throughout these chapters, we have explored the reasoning that shapes medical decisions the factors doctors consider before prescribing, the science behind dosing, the importance of timing, and the consequences that can follow when treatment plans drift from their original design. We have examined the psychological forces that influence adherence and the communication barriers that often stand between patients and clarity. Through real-world stories, we have seen how misunderstanding can quietly undermine care, and how explanation can restore balance.

What emerges is a consistent pattern. When patients understand the "why" behind their treatment, they are better equipped to participate in it. When clinicians understand the realities of their patients' lives, they can design plans that are both effective and sustainable. Neither side carries the full responsibility alone. Effective care lives in the space between knowledge and experience.

This partnership does not require perfection. It does not demand flawless adherence or unwavering certainty. It asks for openness for questions to be asked, for concerns to be voiced, and for limitations to be acknowledged. It allows room for adjustment without silence, and for uncertainty without shame. In that space, trust grows.

Understanding also reshapes accountability. Following a treatment plan becomes less about obedience and more about alignment. Patients are no longer simply complying; they are choosing to engage. When adjustments are needed, they are made through conversation rather than guesswork. This shift transforms care from something imposed into something shared.

The future of healthcare will continue to evolve, bringing new treatments, technologies, and complexities. But no innovation can replace the foundation of clear communication. Information without understanding creates distance. Understanding creates connection. And connection is what allows care to function in the real world.

As you close this book, you are not carrying a list of instructions. You are carrying a framework for thinking a way to interpret medical guidance, to ask better questions, and to recognize when clarity is missing. You are better prepared to engage with your healthcare providers not as a passive recipient, but as an informed participant.

Your health is not a solitary responsibility, nor is it something to be handed over entirely to others. It exists within a partnership built on trust, communication, and shared intention. When you understand the logic behind your care, you strengthen that partnership. And when that partnership is strong, medical instructions stop feeling like constraints and start functioning as what they were always meant to be: support.

This book does not promise certainty. Medicine rarely can. What it offers instead is understanding. And understanding, more than anything else, is what turns care into collaboration and treatment into meaningful action.

About the Author

Dr. Saleem Akram is a pharmacist trained in the clinical sciences, with a professional background rooted in understanding how medicines work and how treatment decisions are made. His Pharm-D training provided extensive exposure to pharmacology, therapeutics, patient care, and the complex considerations that shape prescribing in real clinical settings.

Across his professional experience, **Dr. Akram** observed a recurring pattern: patients often followed medical instructions without fully understanding the reasoning behind them, while clinicians assumed that brief explanations were sufficient. This disconnect subtle but persistent frequently led to confusion, hesitation, and quiet deviations from treatment plans. Rather than viewing these moments as failures, he recognized them as communication gaps.

In parallel with his clinical work, **Dr. Akram** developed a strong focus on medical communication, editing, and publishing. This dual perspective grounded in both healthcare and narrative clarity shaped his approach to patient education. He believes that scientific accuracy alone is not enough; medical knowledge must be communicated in a way that respects how people think, decide, and live.

The Logic of Healing reflects this philosophy. Drawing on clinical training, real-world observation, and structured storytelling, **Dr. Akram** explains the reasoning behind medical decisions without jargon or instruction. His work emphasizes understanding over compliance, partnership over authority, and clarity over complexity.

Dr. Akram continues to advocate for clearer dialogue between patients and healthcare professionals, guided by the conviction that when people understand their care, they are more confident, more engaged, and better equipped to participate meaningfully in their own health decisions.

www.ingramcontent.com/pod-product-compliance
Lightning Source LLC
LaVergne TN
LVHW050939210926
848482LV00013B/678
* 9 7 9 8 2 9 5 5 5 3 7 6 9 *